ALZHEIMER'S (MIND/BRAIN) DIET GUIDE COOKBOOK

NATALIE BROWN

Copyright ©2024.

All rights reserved. No part of this publication may be reproduced, distributed, or transmitted in any form or by any means, including photocopying, recording, or other electronic or mechanical methods, without the prior written permission of the publisher, except in the case of brief quotations embodied in critical reviews and certain other non commercial uses permitted by copyright law

TABLE OF CONTENTS

WHAT IS ALZHEIMER'S DISEASE?

Alzheimer's disease stands as the most prevalent form of dementia, a progressive neurological condition that typically commences with subtle memory lapses and can eventually strip away an individual's ability to engage in conversations and respond to their surroundings. This formidable ailment affects the brain regions responsible for cognition, memory, and language.

Alzheimer's disease (AD) is a neurodegenerative disorder characterized by a gradual decline in cognitive abilities and behavioral functions, significantly impeding both social interactions and occupational activities. It presents as an incurable condition that manifests a prolonged preclinical phase before symptoms become overt, marking its inexorable and relentless progression. Within the intricate landscape of AD, plaques form within the hippocampus—a crucial brain structure integral to memory encoding—as well as in various regions of the cerebral cortex associated with higher-order thinking processes and decision-making.

These plaques, comprised primarily of beta-amyloid protein fragments, have been a focal point in Alzheimer's research, raising questions about their role in the disease. While their presence is a hallmark of Alzheimer's, whether these plaques are the causative agents triggering the disease or merely a byproduct of the underlying pathological process remains an enigma in the scientific realm.

Researchers strive to decipher the intricate mechanisms underlying Alzheimer's pathology, investigating whether these plaques contribute directly to neuronal damage and cognitive decline or if they represent an auxiliary outcome in a more complex cascade of events. Understanding the intricate interplay between plaques, tau protein tangles, inflammation, genetic predispositions, and other factors remains crucial in unraveling the mysteries of Alzheimer's disease and potentially identifying targets for therapeutic intervention. As investigations persist, advancements in research hold promise for unraveling the complexities of this debilitating condition, offering hope for improved diagnostic methods and eventually, effective treatments. Alzheimer's disease is a progressive neurologic disorder that causes the brain to shrink (atrophy) and brain cells to die. Alzheimer's disease is the most common cause of dementia — a continuous decline in thinking, behavioral and social skills that affects a person's ability to function independently.

Approximately 5.8 million people in the United States age 65 and older live with Alzheimer's disease. Of those, 80% are 75 years old and older. Out of the approximately 50 million people worldwide with dementia, between 60% and 70% are estimated to have Alzheimer's disease.

The early signs of the disease include forgetting recent events or conversations. As the disease progresses, a person with Alzheimer's disease will develop severe memory impairment and lose the ability to carry out everyday tasks.

Medications may temporarily improve or slow progression of symptoms. These treatments can sometimes help people with Alzheimer's disease maximize function and maintain independence for a time. Different programs and services can help support people with Alzheimer's disease and their caregivers.

There is no treatment that cures Alzheimer's disease or alters the disease process in the brain. In advanced stages of the disease, complications from severe loss of brain function — such as dehydration, malnutrition or infection — result in death.

SYMPTOMS OF ALZHEIMER'S DISEASE

Symptoms of Alzheimer's disease encompass a range of cognitive and behavioral changes, with memory loss serving as the hallmark indicator of the condition. In the early stages, individuals may struggle to recall recent events or conversations, but as the disease progresses, these memory impairments intensify, often accompanied by the emergence of other distressing symptoms.

Initially, individuals with Alzheimer's may perceive their difficulty remembering things and organizing thoughts. However, it's often the observations of family members or close friends that highlight the worsening nature of these symptoms. The disease precipitates significant brain changes, predominantly affecting:

MEMORY:

While occasional memory lapses are normal, the memory loss associated with Alzheimer's persists and worsens, severely impacting an individual's ability to function both at home and in professional settings. People with Alzheimer's may repeatedly ask the same questions, forget recent conversations or appointments, misplace belongings frequently, get lost in familiar places, and eventually struggle to recall the names of family members or everyday objects. They may also encounter difficulty finding the right words to express thoughts or engage in conversations.

THINKING AND REASONING:

Alzheimer's disrupts concentration and abstract thinking abilities, making multitasking particularly challenging. Tasks that involve managing finances, balancing checkbooks, or handling bills on time become increasingly difficult. Ultimately, individuals with Alzheimer's may face issues recognizing and managing numbers, impacting their ability to handle everyday situations that require numerical reasoning.

JUDGMENT AND DECISION-MAKING:

The disease impairs the ability to make sound judgments in day-to-day situations. This can manifest in poor choices in social interactions or inappropriate attire for the weather. Responding effectively to commonplace problems like burnt food on the stove or unexpected driving situations becomes more challenging.

PERFORMING FAMILIAR TASKS:

Activities that once were routine and required sequential steps, such as planning and cooking meals or playing familiar games, become progressively difficult as the disease advances. Individuals may eventually forget how to perform basic tasks like dressing or bathing.

CHANGES IN PERSONALITY AND BEHAVIOR:

Alzheimer's-related brain changes can influence mood and behavior. Individuals may experience depression, apathy, social withdrawal, mood swings, distrust in others, irritability, changes in sleep patterns, wandering, loss of inhibitions, and occasionally, develop delusions.

While these symptoms progress, certain skills may remain preserved for extended periods despite worsening cognitive decline. These preserved abilities, such as reading, listening to books, storytelling, singing, listening to music, dancing, drawing, or engaging in crafts, often persist due to the involvement of brain regions affected later in the disease progression.

Seeking medical advice is crucial if memory concerns or cognitive changes arise. Conditions other than Alzheimer's, some treatable, can also cause memory loss or dementia-like symptoms. Consulting with a doctor for a comprehensive assessment and diagnosis is essential for proper management and care.

The precise causes of Alzheimer's disease remain a subject of ongoing research. At its core, abnormalities in brain proteins disrupt neuronal function, triggering a cascade of toxic events that damage and eventually cause the death of neurons. Scientists believe that a combination of genetic, lifestyle, and environmental factors affect the brain over time, contributing to the development of the disease.

In the majority of cases, Alzheimer's results from a complex interplay of these factors rather than a single cause. Rarely, specific genetic changes virtually guarantee a person will develop the disease, typically leading to its onset in middle age. The damage often commences in the brain region responsible for memory, years before symptoms emerge. As the disease progresses, neuronal loss spreads in a somewhat predictable pattern to other brain regions, resulting in significant brain shrinkage in advanced stages.

Researchers focus their investigations on two primary proteins implicated in Alzheimer's disease:

1. **Plaques:** Fragments of beta-amyloid protein cluster together, forming amyloid plaques, which disrupt cell-to-cell communication and are toxic to neurons.

2. **Tangles:** Tau proteins, crucial for a neuron's internal support and nutrient transport, undergo structural changes and form neurofibrillary tangles. These tangles disrupt the transport system within neurons and are harmful to cells. Understanding the roles and interactions of these proteins is central to unraveling the intricate mechanisms of Alzheimer's disease and exploring potential avenues for effective treatments or interventions.

RISK FACTORS OF ALZEIMHER

Age

Increasing age is the greatest known risk factor for Alzheimer's disease. Alzheimer's is not a part of normal aging, but as you grow older the likelihood of developing Alzheimer's disease increases.

One study, for example, found that annually there were four new diagnoses per 1,000 people ages 65 to 74, 32 new diagnoses per 1,000 people ages 75 to 84, and 76 new diagnoses per 1,000 people age 85 and older.

Family history and genetics

Your risk of developing Alzheimer's is somewhat higher if a first-degree relative — your parent or sibling — has the disease. Most genetic mechanisms of Alzheimer's among families remain largely unexplained, and the genetic factors are likely complex.

One better understood genetic factor is a form of the apolipoprotein E gene (APOE). A variation of the gene, APOE e4, increases the risk of Alzheimer's disease. Approximately 25% to 30% of the population carries an APOE e4 allele, but not everyone with this variation of the gene develops the disease.

Scientists have identified rare changes (mutations) in three genes that virtually guarantee a person who inherits one of them will develop Alzheimer's. But these mutations account for less than 1% of people with Alzheimer's disease.

Down syndrome

Many people with Down syndrome develop Alzheimer's disease. This is likely related to having three copies of chromosome 21 — and subsequently three copies of the gene for the protein that leads to the creation of beta-amyloid. Signs and symptoms of Alzheimer's tend to appear 10 to 20 years earlier in people with Down syndrome than they do for the general population.

Sex

There appears to be little difference in risk between men and women, but, overall, there are more women with the disease because they generally live longer than men.

Mild cognitive impairment

Mild cognitive impairment (MCI) is a decline in memory or other thinking skills that is greater than normal for a person's age, but the decline doesn't prevent a person from functioning in social or work environments.

People who have MCI have a significant risk of developing dementia. When the primary MCI deficit is memory, the condition is more likely to progress to dementia due to Alzheimer's disease. A diagnosis of MCI encourages a greater focus on healthy lifestyle changes, developing strategies to make up for memory loss and scheduling regular doctor appointments to monitor symptoms.

Head trauma

People who've had a severe head trauma have a greater risk of Alzheimer's disease. Several large studies found that in people age 50 years or older who had a traumatic brain injury (TBI), the risk of dementia and Alzheimer's disease increased. The risk increases in people with more-severe and multiple TBIs. Some studies indicate that the risk may be greatest within the first six months to two years after the TBI.

Air pollution

Studies in animals have indicated that air pollution particulates can speed degeneration of the nervous system. And human studies have found that air pollution exposure — particularly from traffic exhaust and burning wood — is associated with greater dementia risk.

Excessive alcohol consumption

Drinking large amounts of alcohol has long been known to cause brain changes. Several large studies and reviews found that alcohol use disorders were linked to an increased risk of dementia, particularly early-onset dementia.

Poor sleep patterns

Research has shown that poor sleep patterns, such as difficulty falling asleep or staying asleep, are associated with an increased risk of Alzheimer's disease.

Lifestyle and heart health

Research has shown that the same risk factors associated with heart disease may also increase the risk of Alzheimer's disease. These include:

- Lack of exercise
- Obesity
- Smoking or exposure to secondhand smoke
- High blood pressure
- High cholesterol
- Poorly controlled type 2 diabetes

These factors can all be modified. Therefore, changing lifestyle habits can to some degree alter your risk. For example, regular exercise and a healthy low-fat diet rich in fruits and vegetables are associated with a decreased risk of developing Alzheimer's disease.

Lifelong learning and social engagement

Studies have found an association between lifelong involvement in mentally and socially stimulating activities and a reduced risk of Alzheimer's disease. Low education levels — less than a high school education — appear to be a risk factor for Alzheimer's disease.

Complications

Memory and language loss, impaired judgment and other cognitive changes caused by Alzheimer's can complicate treatment for other health conditions. A person with Alzheimer's disease may not be able to:

- Communicate that he or she is experiencing pain
- Explain symptoms of another illness
- Follow a prescribed treatment plan

- Explain medication side effects

As Alzheimer's disease progresses to its last stages, brain changes begin to affect physical functions, such as swallowing, balance, and bowel and bladder control. These effects can increase vulnerability to additional health problems such as:

- Inhaling food or liquid into the lungs (aspiration)
- Flu, pneumonia and other infections
- Falls
- Fractures
- Bedsores
- Malnutrition or dehydration
- Constipation or diarrhea
- Dental problems such as mouth sores or tooth decay

Prevention

Alzheimer's disease is not a preventable condition. However, a number of lifestyle risk factors for Alzheimer's can be modified. Evidence suggests that changes in diet, exercise and habits — steps to reduce the risk of cardiovascular disease — may also lower your risk of developing Alzheimer's disease and other disorders that cause dementia. Heart-healthy lifestyle choices that may reduce the risk of Alzheimer's include the following:

- Exercising regularly
- Eating a diet of fresh produce, healthy oils and foods low in saturated fat such as a Mediterranean diet
- Following treatment guidelines to manage high blood pressure, diabetes and high cholesterol
- Asking your doctor for help to quit smoking if you smoke

Studies have shown that preserved thinking skills later in life and a reduced risk of Alzheimer's disease are associated with participating in social events, reading, dancing, playing board games, creating art, playing an instrument, and other activities that require mental and social engagement.

Diagnosis

An important part of diagnosing Alzheimer's disease includes being able to explain your symptoms, as well as perspective from a close family member or friend about symptoms and their impact on daily life. Additionally, a diagnosis of Alzheimer's disease is based on tests your doctor administers to assess memory and thinking skills.

Laboratory and imaging tests can rule out other potential causes or help the doctor better identify the disease causing dementia symptoms.

But Alzheimer's disease is only diagnosed with complete certainty after death, when microscopic examination of the brain reveals the characteristic plaques and tangles.

Tests

A diagnostic work-up would likely include the following tests:

Physical and neurological exam

Your doctor will perform a physical exam and likely assess overall neurological health by testing the following:

- Reflexes
- Muscle tone and strength
- Ability to get up from a chair and walk across the room
- Sense of sight and hearing
- Coordination
- Balance

Lab tests

Blood tests may help your doctor rule out other potential causes of memory loss and confusion, such as a thyroid disorder or vitamin deficiencies.

Mental status and neuropsychological testing

Your doctor may give you a brief mental status test to assess memory and other thinking skills. Longer forms of neuropsychological testing may provide additional details about mental function compared with people of a similar age and education level. These tests can help establish a diagnosis and serve as a starting point to track the progression of symptoms in the future.

Brain imaging

Images of the brain are now used chiefly to pinpoint visible abnormalities related to conditions other than Alzheimer's disease — such as strokes, trauma or tumors — that may cause cognitive change. New imaging applications — currently used primarily in major medical centers or in clinical trials — may enable doctors to detect specific brain changes caused by Alzheimer's.

Imaging of brain structures include the following:

- Magnetic resonance imaging (MRI). MRI uses radio waves and a strong magnetic field to produce detailed images of the brain. While they may show brain shrinkage of brain regions associated with Alzheimer's disease, MRI scans also rule out other conditions. An MRI is generally preferred to a CT scan for the evaluation of dementia.
- Computerized tomography (CT). A CT scan, a specialized X-ray technology, produces cross-sectional images (slices)

of your brain. It's usually used to rule out tumors, strokes and head injuries.

- Imaging of disease processes can be performed with positron emission tomography (PET). During a PET scan, a low-level radioactive tracer is injected into the blood to reveal a particular feature in the brain. PET imaging may include the following:
- Fluorodeoxyglucose (FDG) PET scans show areas of the brain in which nutrients are poorly metabolized. Identifying patterns of degeneration — areas of low metabolism — can help distinguish between Alzheimer's disease and other types of dementia.
- Amyloid PET imaging can measure the burden of amyloid deposits in the brain. This imaging is primarily used in research but may be used if a person has unusual or very early onset of dementia symptoms.
- Tau PET imaging, which measures the burden of neurofibrillary tangles in the brain, is generally used in the research setting.

In special circumstances, such as rapidly progressive dementia, dementia with atypical features or early-onset dementia, other tests may be used to measure abnormal beta-amyloid and tau in the cerebrospinal fluid.

ALZHEIMER'S DIET RECIPES

BRAIN CHARGE FRUITY SMOOTHIE

INGREDIENTS

- 2 Mango Peeled and chopped
- 100 grams Raspberries Fresh or frozen
- 1/2 Avocado Peeled and chopped
- 1 tablespoon Chia seeds
- 1 tablespoon Flax seed also known as linseed
- 200 millilitres Coconut water

INSTRUCTIONS

1. Place all the ingredients in your food blender or Nutribullet and smoosh until smooth.

ALMOND-OAT NOG

INGREDIENTS

- 1 quart almond milk (unsweetened unflavored), store-bought or homemade

- ½ cup oats old-fashioned or quick
- 1 tablespoon pure maple syrup
- 1 teaspoon pure vanilla extract
- ½ teaspoon ground cinnamon
- ¼ teaspoon ground nutmeg plus more for serving, preferably freshly ground
- ¼ teaspoon ground cardamom
- ¼ teaspoon kosher salt
- ¼ teaspoon pure almond extract optional
- Rum optional

INSTRUCTIONS

1. Combine almond milk, oats, maple syrup, vanilla, cinnamon, nutmeg, cardamom, salt, and almond extract (if using) in a blender. Pulse for a few seconds to distribute the oats, and let sit for about 10 minutes so that they soften.

2. Blend on high until completely smooth and frothy, about 1 minute. To serve warm, pour into a small pot and heat gently over low heat, being careful not to bring to a boil. To serve cold, chill in the refrigerator. Just before serving, sprinkle

with more nutmeg. Spike with a dash of rum, if using.

DOUBLE CHOCOLATE AND PISTACHIO BISCOTTI

INGREDIENTS

- 2 cups almond flour plus more for dusting
- ¾ cup natural cacao powder
- ¾ teaspoon baking powder
- ¾ teaspoon baking soda
- ½ teaspoon kosher salt
- 3 large eggs at room temperature
- ¾ cup coconut palm sugar
- 1 teaspoon pure vanilla extract
- 1 teaspoon almond extract
- 1 cup raw pistachios toasted (see Note)
- ½ cup dark chocolate chips
- For the glaze:
- ½ cup dark chocolate chips
- 1 teaspoon extra virgin olive oil

INSTRUCTIONS

1. Preheat the oven to 375°F with a rack set in the center position. Line a rimmed baking sheet with parchment paper or a silicone mat.

2. In a medium bowl, whisk together the flour, cacao powder, baking powder, baking soda, and salt. In a large mixing bowl or the bowl of a standing mixer, beat together the eggs, sugar, and vanilla and almond extracts. Gradually add the dry ingredients until no streaks of flour remain. Fold in the nuts and ½ cup chocolate chips until evenly distributed.

3. Dust your work surface with flour and divide the dough into two equal balls. The dough will be sticky so dust your hands with flour, too. Flatten each half of dough out into a rectangular log that is 10 inches long, 2 ½ inches wide, and 1 inch tall. Transfer the logs to the baking sheet, reshape if needed, and bake until the dough is lightly browned, with cracks on the surface, and springy to the touch, 20 to 25 minutes. Set aside until completely cool, about 15 to 30 minutes depending

on the temperature of your kitchen. Reduce the oven temperature to 300°F.

4. Carefully transfer the logs to a cutting board. Use a serrated knife to slice the cookies straight up and down, about ½-inch thick. Transfer the cookie slices back to the baking sheet and place them standing up. (You can crowd all the cookies onto the same pan or use an additional baking sheet.) Bake until the biscotti are dry to the touch and no longer springy, 25 to 35 minutes.

5. While the biscotti cool, make the chocolate glaze. Place the chocolate chips in a heat-proof bowl over a small pot of boiling water, making sure the water doesn't touch the bottom of the bowl. When the chocolate is melted, whisk in the olive oil until you have a smooth glaze. Drizzle over the cooled biscotti and let sit until the glaze has set.

6. To store, keep in an airtight container for up to 3 weeks.

MUSHROOM AND DELICATA SqUASH SOUP WITH FARRO

INGREDIENTS

- 2 tablespoons extra virgin olive oil
- 2 large celery stalks finely chopped (about ¾ cup), leaves torn and reserved for garnish
- 2 large shallots finely chopped (about ⅔ cup)
- 1 teaspoon kosher salt divided
- 2 large garlic cloves coarsely chopped (about 1 tablespoon)
- ½ teaspoon freshly ground black pepper
- 1 pound mixed fresh mushrooms such as cremini, button, maitake, oyster, and shiitake, trimmed and roughly chopped (about 6 cups total)
- 1 medium mediumdelicata squash halved lengthwise, seeded, and cut into half moons
- ½ cup semi-pearled farro
- 8 cups vegetable stock or water
- 2 tablespoons white miso paste
- 1 large lemon juiced and zested

- Flaky salt optional

INSTRUCTIONS

1. Heat the oil over medium heat in a large pot. Add the celery, shallot, and ½ teaspoon each salt and pepper. Cook over medium heat, stirring often, until the vegetables are soft and translucent, 8 to 10 minutes. Stir in the garlic and cook for 1 minute more.

2. Add the mushrooms and cook, stirring occasionally, until soft and starting to soften and release their liquid, 6 to 8 minutes. Stir in the squash, farro, stock, and the remaining ½ teaspoon salt. Bring to a boil, then reduce to a simmer and cook until you can easily pierce the squash with the tip of a knife and the farro is tender but chewy, 20 to 25 minutes.

3. Use a fork to stir 2 tablespoons of the warm broth with the miso paste in a small bowl to make a smooth paste. Stir the miso mixture, lemon juice and zest into the soup. Continue to cook until warmed through.

4. Divide the soup between bowls and sprinkle with the celery leaves and flaky salt, if using, plus more fresh ground black pepper, if you like.

BETTER-FOR-YOU EGGPLANT PARM

INGREDIENTS

- 1 large eggplant cut into ½-inch rounds
- 1 ¼ teaspoons kosher salt divided
- ¼ cup extra virgin olive oil plus more for cooking the eggplant
- 3 large garlic cloves, minced about 1 tablespoon
- 2 cups cherry tomatoes
- ½ cup white wine
- 1 large egg
- 2 tablespoons water
- 1 cup whole-wheat panko or regular bread crumbs
- 2 cups Lemony Cashew Ricotta or store-bought almond or cashew ricotta, or part-skim or low-fat ricotta
- ¼ cup grated Parmesan optional
- fresh basil leaves torn

INSTRUCTIONS

1. Place the eggplant slices onto a rimmed baking sheet and sprinkle both sides with salt (about 1 teaspoon total). Let sit while you make the sauce.

2. Combine ¼ cup olive oil, garlic, tomatoes, and ¼ teaspoon salt in a medium saucepan over medium-low heat, stirring often to make sure the garlic doesn't burn. When the tomatoes start to split, after about 10 minutes, press on them with the back of a spoon, add the wine, and simmer over medium-low heat until you have a loose sauce, another 10-15 minutes. Set aside.

3. Set out two pie plates. Beat the egg with 2 tablespoons of water and pour onto one pie plate. Add the bread crumbs to the other. Blot the eggplant slices thoroughly with paper towels and dip each slice in the egg/water mixture to coat. Dredge in the bread crumbs, pressing down so they adhere. Place back on the baking sheet and continue until all your eggplant slices are coated.

4. In a large nonstick skillet, heat 2 tablespoons of olive oil over medium heat. Add as many eggplant slices as will fit with a little room on each side, and pan-fry until the bottom is golden brown, 5 to 7 minutes. Using long tongs, flip each slice and cook until golden on the other side. Place the eggplant back on the baking sheet while you cook as many slices as you want, adding more oil if needed.

5. To serve, pour a ladle-full of sauce into shallow bowls. Add an eggplant slice, dollop with about 2 tablespoons of ricotta, and top with another piece of eggplant. Finish with a light dusting of grated Parmesan, if you wish, and fresh basil.

TURKEY PARM BURGERS

INGREDIENTS

- 1 cup raw walnuts
- ¼ cup nutritional yeast or grated Parmesan cheese
- 2 tablespoons white miso paste
- 1 medium garlic clove
- 1/4 teaspoon red pepper flakes
- 1 pound ground turkey 93% to 98% lean
- 1 medium zucchini (about 7 ounces) grated and squeezed dry to yield about 1 cup
- ½ cup plant-based mayo from a jar
- 1 to 2 tablespoon harissa or other spice paste
- 4 whole-grain buns or serve on a bed of greens
- 1 large tomato sliced
- microgreens

INSTRUCTIONS

1. Combine the walnuts, nutritional yeast or grated Parmesan, miso paste, garlic, and red pepper flakes in the bowl of a food

processor. Pulse until the mixture forms small, uniform crumbles, like wet sand or coarsely grated Parmesan cheese. Scrape into a large bowl with the turkey and zucchini. Using your hands or a large fork, mix until just combined. Press into 4 patties, each about 1-inch thick.

2. When ready to grill, light the grill with a high heat zone and a medium heat zone (about 350°F). Clean the grill well with a stiff brush and coat the grates with oil. Place the burgers in the medium heat zone and grill until lightly brown and cooked through and an instant read thermometer inserted into the center of the burger reads 165°F, 8 to 10 minutes on each side.

3. For the spicy mayo, stir together the mayo and harissa; set aside. Warm the buns, if using, on the medium hot side of the grill a few minutes before the burgers are done.

4. Serve the burgers on warm buns or a bed of greens topped with a thick slice of tomato, a dollop of spicy mayo, and as many microgreens as you like.

QUINOA CHIA SEED PUDDING WITH GRAPEFRUIT AND POMEGRANATE

INGREDIENTS

- For the pudding:
- ½ cup white or red quinoa, or a mix or 1 cup cooked quinoa
- ¼ cup black chia seeds
- 1½ cups unsweetened, unflavored cashew milk or another plant-based milk
- up to 1 tablespoon pure maple syrup optional
- ½ teaspoon pure vanilla extract
- ¼ teaspoon almond extract
- For the topping:
- 1 grapefruit peeled and cut into segments
- ½ cup pomegranate seeds

INSTRUCTIONS

1. Place the quinoa, 1 cup water, and a pinch of salt in a medium saucepan that has a tight-fitting lid. Bring to a boil over medium-high heat, then reduce the heat to a gentle simmer. Cover and cook until the quinoa has absorbed almost all its

water, 15 to 20 minutes. Remove from the heat, cover, and let the quinoa steam for at least 5 minutes or until you are ready to serve.

2. Combine the chia seeds and milk in a small bowl and refrigerate until plump, about 1 hour. Fold in the quinoa, up to 1 tablespoon of maple syrup, if using, and the vanilla and almonds extracts.

3. To serve, divide pudding between 4 jars. Top each with grapefruit pieces and pomegranate arils.

4. Serve right away or keep, tightly covered, in the refrigerator for up to 5 days.

CRANBERRY CHUTNEY

INGREDIENTS

- 3 cups fresh cranberries
- ½ cup water
- 3 tablespoons date syrup or honey
- 1 teaspoon small jalapeno chile seeds removed, finely diced + 1 to sprinkle on top
- ½ teaspoon ground coriander
- ½ teaspoon ground turmeric

- ¼ teaspoon kosher salt

INSTRUCTIONS

1. Combine the cranberries, water, date syrup, chiles, coriander, turmeric, and salt in a medium saucepan and bring to a boil over medium-high heat.
2. When the cranberries start to pop, reduce the heat to a gentle simmer.
3. Cook, stirring often, until the sauce coats the back of a spoon, 15 to 20 minutes. Sprinkle with more jalapeño before serving.

CHAI-SPICED CRANBERRY APPLE COMPOTE

INGREDIENTS

- 1 cup water
- 1 chai tea bag
- 3 cups fresh cranberries
- 1 cups large tart apple such as a Granny Smith or Honeycrisp, ½-inch dice (about 1½| TK g)
- 2 tablespoons date syrup or honey

- ½ teaspoon ground cardamom
- ¼ teaspoon kosher salt
- ¼ teaspoon reshly ground black pepper
- ¼ cup candied ginger finely diced + more to sprinkle on top.

INSTRUCTIONS

1. Bring the water to a boil in a medium saucepan, add the tea bag, and turn off the heat. Steep for 5 minutes and discard (or reuse) the tea bag.
2. Add the cranberries, apple, date syrup, cardamom, salt, and freshly ground black pepper to the tea and bring to a boil. When the cranberries start to pop, reduce the heat to a gentle simmer.
3. Cook, stirring often, until the sauce coats the back of a spoon, 15 to 20 minutes. Stir in the candied ginger and sprinkle a few teaspoons on top.

PUMPKIN BLUEBERRY MUFFINS

INGREDIENTS

- 1 cup oat flour
- 1 cup almond flour
- ¼ cup hemp seeds (also called hemp hearts) plus 1 tablespoon to top the muffins
- 2 teaspoons baking powder
- 1 tablespoon ground flaxseeds
- 1 teaspoon ground cinnamon
- ½ teaspoon kosher salt
- 1 cup pumpkin puree from a can
- ⅔ cup coconut palm sugar
- ½ cup extra virgin olive oil
- 1 teaspoon pure vanilla extract
- 1 teaspoon almond extract
- 2 large eggs
- 2 cups blueberries fresh or frozen (don't defrost)

INSTRUCTIONS

1. Preheat your oven to 350°F. Line a 12-cup muffin tin with paper liners and set aside.
2. In a large bowl, whisk together the oat and almond flours, ¼ cup of the hemp hearts, the baking powder, ground flaxseed, cinnamon, and ½ teaspoon salt; set aside.
3. In a separate large bowl, whisk together the pumpkin, sugar, olive oil, vanilla, and almond extracts. Whisk in the eggs one at a time. Fold the dry ingredients into the wet ones until just combined.
4. Gently fold 1⅓ cups of the blueberries into the muffin batter. Divide the batter evenly between the muffin cups.
5. Divide the remaining ⅔ cup blueberries over the tops of the muffins and gently press them into the batter. Sprinkle with the additional tablespoon of hemp hearts.
6. Bake for 38 to 42 minutes for standard muffins, or until a cake tester or small wooden skewer inserted into muffins

comes out clean. For mini muffins, check for doneness starting at 32 minutes.

7. These muffins are best the day they are made or the next day. Warm day-old muffins in the oven at 300ºF for 10 minutes. To freeze, wrap in plastic wrap and store in the freezer for up to 6 months.

DRIED FIG AND OLIVE TAPENADE

INGREDIENTS

- 1 cup dried figs packed
- ½ cup black olives pitted
- ½ cup green olives pitted
- 2 to 3 tablespoons extra virgin olive oil
- 1 teaspoon minced fresh rosemary plus a sprig for garnish
- 1 tablespoon balsamic vinegar
- 2 teaspoons capers rinsed of salt
- To serve:
- 3 to 4 radishes, with greens thinly sliced
- 3 to 4 spring turnips, with greens thinly sliced
- whole-grain crackers

INSTRUCTIONS

1. Use scissors to snip off the stems of the figs.
2. Place the figs, olives, olive oil, rosemary, vinegar, and capers in the bowl of a food processor. Pulse until it turns into a chunky spread, adding more oil if needed.
3. Scrape the tapenade into a serving bowl topped with the sprig of rosemary. Serve with whole-grain crackers and sliced fresh vegetables, such as radishes and spring turnips.

CRISPY TAHINI RICE BARS

INGREDIENTS

- 1 cup raw cashews
- ⅓ cup raw sesame seeds
- 1 cup soft dates pitted and chopped (about 14 Medjool dates) or pulsed in a food processor
- ¼ cup honey

- ½ cup tahini well-stirred and at room temperature
- 2 cups crispy brown rice cereal
- 1 teaspoon freshly grated ginger
- 1 teaspoon extra virgin olive oil
- ½ teaspoon kosher salt

INSTRUCTIONS

1. Preheat your oven to 325° F. Place the cashews in an 8 x 8-inch square baking dish (such as a brownie pan) and roast for 10 minutes, or until they are a shade darker and have a toasty aroma. Transfer to a large mixing bowl.

2. Place the sesame seeds in the same baking dish and toast in the oven for 3 to 5 minutes, or until just starting to turn golden. Add to the bowl with the cashews.

3. In a small saucepan over low heat, warm the dates, honey, and tahini, stirring to combine. When the tahini mixture is bubbling gently, turn off the heat and stir in the ginger and salt. Pour over the cashews and sesame seeds and fold to combine until evenly coated. Gently fold

in the rice cereal, stirring until evenly coated but taking care not to crush it.

4. Coat the baking dish with the oil (using an oven mitt if the pan is still hot) and line it with parchment paper so there's a few inches of overhang on 2 sides. Scrape the mixture into the baking dish and press firmly into an even layer. It helps to use the flat bottom of a measuring cup or a metal spatula (spray with olive oil first) to really compact the bars into the pan.

5. Bake for 20 to 22 minutes, or until the edges are golden brown and the center is firm. Remove from the oven and let cool in the pan. Chill in the refrigerator for 45 minutes before cutting into bars.

6. Lift the parchment to transfer the bars to a cutting board. Cut into 25 1-by-1-inch bars. (A serrated knife works well for this.)

CITRUSY COD PACKETS WITH ZUCCHINI AND QUINOA

INGREDIENTS

- 4 4-ounce pieces boneless, skin-on cod filets about 1-inch thick
- ½ cup fresh orange juice plus 2 tablespoons zest
- ⅓ cup fresh lemon juice plus 2 tablespoons zest
- 1 teaspoon kosher salt divided, plus more to taste
- 1 ¾ cups water
- 1 cup quinoa rinsed
- 1 medium zucchini spiralized, about 3 cups
- 3 tablespoons extra virgin olive oil plus more for coating the paper
- 2 medium garlic cloves thinly sliced
- ¼ teaspoon freshly ground black pepper
- 2 blood oranges very thinly sliced into half-moons
- Flaky salt to finish
- Cilantro leaves optional

INSTRUCTIONS

1. Preheat your oven to 400°F.
2. Place the cod in a 1-quart-size rimmed baking dish and pour the juices over them. Flip the fish over a few times so that the pieces are coated with the marinade, then place skin-side down. Sprinkle with ½ teaspoon of the salt, cover, and place in the fridge for at least 20 minutes and up to 1 hour.
3. While the cod marinates, cook the quinoa. Combine the water and quinoa in a medium saucepan with a tight-fitting lid and bring to a boil. Reduce the heat to a low simmer and cook for 15 minutes. Remove the pot from the heat, covered, and let it sit for 10 more minutes. Fluff with a fork when ready to use.
4. Meanwhile, place the zucchini in a medium bowl with the orange and lemon zests, oil, garlic, pepper, and the remaining ½ teaspoon salt. Toss well to coat and set aside.

5. To assemble the packets, lay out four 10-by-14-inch pieces of parchment paper. Fold each sheet in half, forming a 7-by-10-inch rectangle. Use scissors to cut out a half-moon as big as the paper allows. Unfold the half moon of paper into a circle. Brush one half with olive oil, and divide the quinoa, vegetables, and fish pieces (skin-side down) between the four oiled halves. Top each piece of cod with 3 to 4 blood orange slices. Drizzle a few spoonfuls of marinade over the fish.

6. To seal the packets, fold the top half of parchment over the fish and align the edges. Starting at one corner, fold over about ½-inch of the edge 3 times, pressing down to make a crisp crease after each fold. Continue to work your way around the edge of the packet, making overlapping, pleat-like folds, always pressing firmly and creasing the edge so the folds hold. When you get to the end of the paper, twist it into a tail to prevent the liquid from seeping out. If necessary, make a second fold wherever there doesn't appear to be a tight seal.

When finished, your packet will look like
a large calzone.

7. Place the packets on a rimmed baking
sheet. Bake for 15 minutes. The paper
will darken and puff up as the packet fills
with steam. Cooking time will depend on
the thickness of your fish; allow a few
more minutes if your filets are more than
1-inch thick.

8. To serve, transfer the packets to a plate.
Using scissors or a sharp knife, slit open
the lids of the packets and fold the paper
back. Sprinkle with flaky salt and top
with cilantro leaves, if using.

CREAMY RED PEPPER SAUCE

INGREDIENTS

- 1 cup raw cashews soaked in very hot tap
water for 15 minutes
- 1 large garlic clove
- 1 cup roasted and peeled sweet red
peppers (from a jar drained)
- 1 tablespoon chopped canned chipotles in
adobo

INSTRUCTIONS

2. Drain the cashews, reserving ½ cup of the soaking water.
3. Combine the cashews and ¼ cup of the soaking water in a blender with the remaining ingredients. Blend on high until smooth.
4. Add more of the cashew soaking water, teaspoon by teaspoon, if needed to achieve a spreadable consistency.
5. Taste, blend in another small piece of chipotle pepper if you prefer more spice. Scrape into a jar.

CRISPY CAULIFLOWER TACOS WITH A CREAMY RED PEPPER SAUCE

INGREDIENTS

- 1 small head of cauliflower about 1½ pounds
- 2 teaspoons chili powder
- ½ teaspoon kosher salt
- 1 tablespoon avocado or extra virgin olive oil
- ¼ cup water

- For the Tacos
- ½ cup Creamy Red Pepper Sauce recipe follows
- 4 Corn tortillas warmed
- 1 cup sugar snap peas sliced thin on the bias
- Cilantro leaves for scrving
- Crumbled feta cheese for serving
- ¼ cup pickled jalapeño peppers
- 1 lime cut into 4 wedges

INSTRUCTIONS

1. Wash and trim the cauliflower, removing any outer leaves. Using a knife, separate the head in half from the top to the stem. Slice into 3-by-3-inch pieces, each about ½-inch thick. (Slicing the cauliflower creates a flat surface to enable a crispy exterior, and keep them from falling out of your taco. It's fine to just break into florets if you prefer.) Toss in a bowl with the chili powder and salt.
2. To cook the cauliflower, heat a large nonstick skillet (that has a tight-fitting lid) over medium heat. Add the oil, and when

it starts to shimmer add the cauliflower pieces, separating them so they do not touch. Once they become brown and crispy on one side, after about 3 minutes, flip them over. Cook until brown and crispy, then carefully pour the water into the skillet and cover. Remove from the heat and let the cauliflower steam in the pan for 1 to 2 minutes, or until easily pierced with a knife.

3. To build your tacos, divide the red pepper sauce, cauliflower, sugar snaps, and jalapenos between the tortillas. Top with cilantro, feta, and a couple pickled jalapeños. Serve each plate with a lime wedge.

CREAMY KALE SOUP

INGREDIENTS

- 1 tablespoon avocado or olive oil
- 1 large onion chopped
- 1 small sweet potato peeled and chopped
- 1 bunch kale stems removed, chopped
- 1 ta fresh rosemary plus more for garnish
- 1 cup vegetable stock

- 2 cups plain, unsweetened almond milk
- 1/2 teaspoon salt
- freshly cracked black pepper to taste
- 1/2 cup sliced almonds toasted

INSTRUCTIONS

1. In a large pot, heat the oil over medium high heat. Add the onions and stir, and once they start to sizzle, reduce the heat to medium. Stir and cook, reducing the heat to medium-low if they start to stick. Cook for as long as you have time, at least 10 minutes, up to an hour or two.

2. Add the sweet potato, kale, rosemary and stock and raise the heat to medium-high. Bring to a boil, cover and cook for about 10 minutes. When the sweet potato pieces are tender, take off the heat.

3. Transfer the soup to the Vitamix or food processor. If using the processor, puree without adding the almond milk. If using the blender, add the milk and puree. Add the salt and several grinds of pepper, and taste. Add more if needed.

4. Serve in bowls with toasted sliced almonds, and a rosemary sprig.

BRAIN-BOOSTING SALAD

INGREDIENTS

- red onion, diced (1/2)
- Mexican gray squash or zucchini, diced (1)
- cucumber, peeled and diced (1)
- small tomatoes, diced (2)
- sliced red cabbage (1/4 cup)
- celery, sliced (2 stalks)
- corn kernals (2 ears or 1 1/2 cups)
- sea salt (pinch)
- fresh lime juice (1 tbsp.)
- tomatillos, diced (3)
- chopped fresh cilantro (2 tbsp.)
- rinsed and cooked or canned red beans, or 1 cup sauteed tempeh (1 cup)
- sliced Swiss chard leaves (1 cup)

INSTRUCTIONS

1. Mix all ingredients together in a large bowl and allow the salad to marinate for at least 30 minutes but preferably 2 hours.

2. You can forgo this step and eat the salad right away, though the flavors won't be melded quite as much.

3. Options: If you use the tomatillos, peel away the papery part and make sure to wash them before cutting; this removes their sticky outer film and makes them much easier to handle. You can also use frozen corn in this recipe, though it will lack the crispness and sweetness of fresh corn. Want to make this a meal in itself instead of an accompaniment? Add the beans or tempeh and you'll have a delicious dinner in minutes.

BLUEBERRY BRAIN SMOOTHIE & HEALTHY BRAIN FOODS

INGREDIENTS

- 8-10 ounces almond milk preferably homemade
- 3/4 cup blueberries or blackberries
- 1 big handful baby spinach leaves
- 2 teaspoons raw unsweetened cocoa powder optional
- 1 teaspoon cinnamon
- 1 small banana
- 1 scoop protein powder

INSTRUCTIONS

1. Place everything in a blender and blend until smooth. Drink immediately.

RED, WHITE, AND BLUE OVERNIGHT OATS

INGREDIENTS

- ¼ cup old fashioned oats
- 5 strawberries
- ¼ cup almond milk (or any milk)
- 1 6 ounce container plain or vanilla yogurt
- 2 tablespoons shredded coconut
- ¼ cup old fashioned oats
- ½ cup blueberries

- ¼ cup almond milk (or any milk)
- tablespoon shredded coconut, if desired

INSTRUCTIONS

1. Slice strawberries in half.
2. Combine each layer's ingredients in 3 separate bowls (i.e. one red bowl, one white bowl and one blue bowl); stir.
3. Layer each flavor into one jar, cup, or bowl. Top with coconut. Refrigerate.

LEMON BLUEBERRY MUFFINS

INGREDIENTS

- 3 cups whole wheat pastry flour
- 1 cup sugar
- 1 tablespoon baking powder
- ¾ teaspoon salt
- ½ cup (1 stick) butter, softened
- 2 eggs, at room temperature
- ¾ cup milk, at room temperature

INSTRUCTIONS

1. Blend all together and serve

BRAIN BOOSTING SUPER SALAD (WITH LEMON VINAIGRETTE)

INGREDIENTS

LEMON VINAIGRETTE

- ¼ cup olive oil

  - ¼ cup lemon juice fresh
  - ¼ teaspoon lemon zest
  - ½ teaspoon honey or date syrup
  - ½ clove garlic minced
  - ⅛ teaspoon salt and pepper to taste

SALAD

  - 1 medium avocado
  - 1 cup broccoli
  - ¼ cup blueberries
  - ¼ cup raspberries
  - ¼ cup blackberries
  - 2 medium plum
  - 2 medium nectarine
  - ¼ cup walnuts chopped

INSTRUCTIONS

LEMON VINAIGRETTE

1. Add all the vinaigrette ingredients to a small bowl.
2. Whisk until everything is combined. Refrigerate until you're ready to use.

SALAD

1. Wash and dry the fruit just before you make the salad.
2. Cut the avocado, nectarines, plums, and broccoli into bite-size pieces and divide them between two bowls.
3. Equally, add the remaining ingredients to the bowls.
4. Toss with salad dressing just before serving.
5. Refrigerate any leftover salad dressing.

MEDITERRANEAN BAKED COD

INGREDIENTS

- 220 g White Fish cod, halibut
- 1 Red Onion small
- 70 g Cherry Tomatoes ½ cup
- 60 g Olives Kalamata or others
- 1 tbsp Lemon Juice
- 3 Garlic Cloves

INSTRUCTIONS

1. Preheat the oven to 180C
2. Chop 1 small red onion, 3 cloves of garlic, and halve cherry tomatoes
3. Pour 3tbsp of olive oil into an oven-proof dish and add garlic
4. Place white fish inside the dish, season with salt and pepper.
5. Combine olives, onion, and tomatoes with dried herbs, salt, pepper, and a squeeze of lemon juice
6. Cover the fish with veg and bake for 20mins
7. Topped with freshly chopped parsley

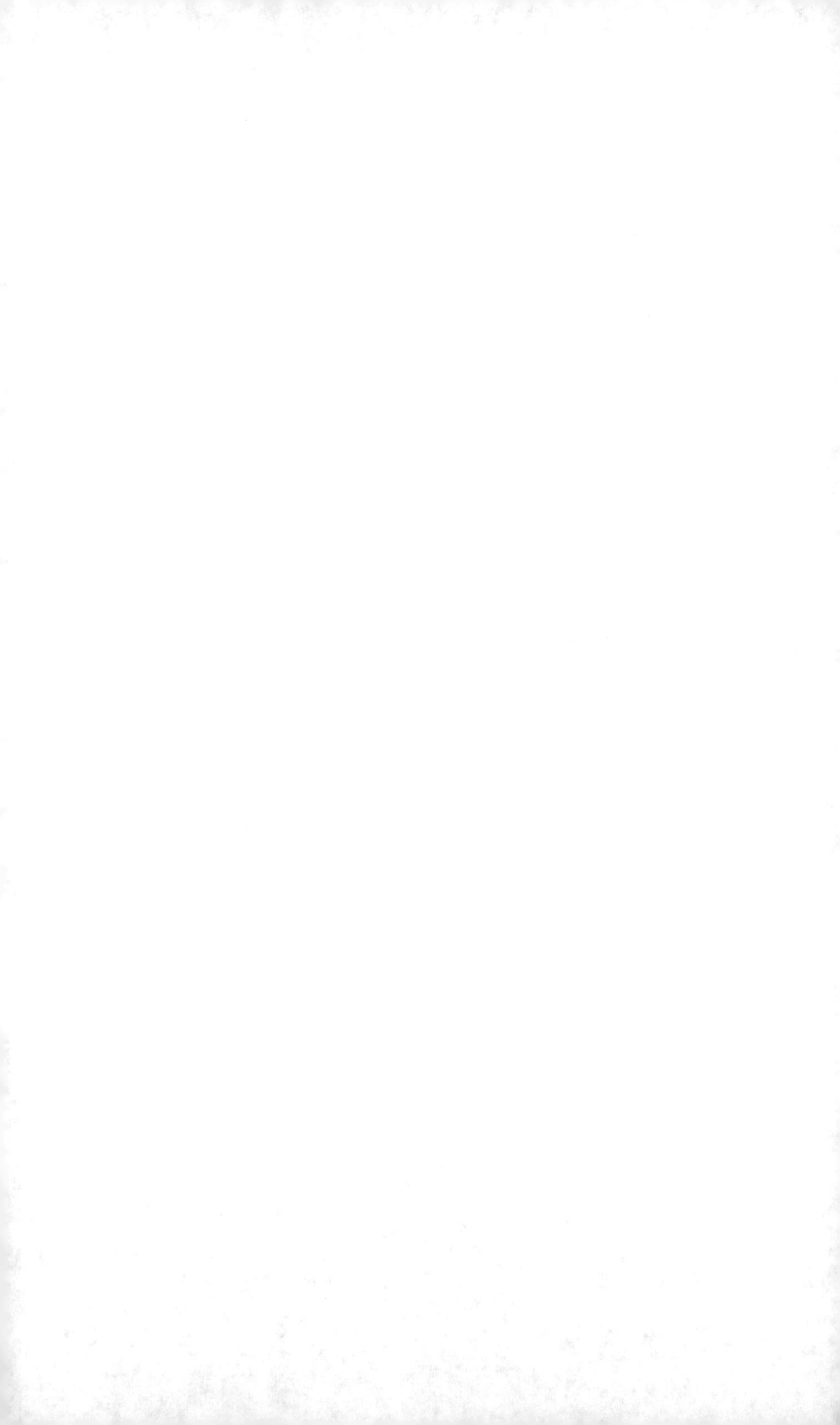